I0844250

Detox and Train

Fitness and Nutritional Reboot for a Healthier You

Table of Contents

Chapter 1. Introduction

Dust off your gym shoes and wave goodbye to unhealthy habits because it's time for a full body reboot! Our Special Report on "Detox and Train: Fitness and Nutritional Reboot for a Healthier You" is your ticket to a revitalized, radiant, and healthier version of you. This comprehensive guide homely amalgamates hit-the-mark fitness regimes and balanced nutritional charts, tailored for both, fitness novices and seasoned athletes. This reader-friendly analysis, based on sound science, will help you understand the connection between detoxification and training; empower you to make informed decisions about your diet and fitness strategies; and ultimately, steer you onto the path of long-term wellness. All that in a vibrant, easy-to-understand way that transforms your incremental changes into monumental health gains. Don't let this opportunity slip away – invest in a fitter, healthier, and happier YOU by snapping up this report today!

Chapter 2. Understanding Detoxification: The Science and Myths

Let's get started on our engaging journey into the fascinating realm of detoxification – a process that is often misunderstood, but regardless, plays a fundamental role in our overall health and well-being.

2.1. The Basics of Detoxification

Our body is a complex ecosystem that constantly interacts with the world around it: with what we eat, drink, breathe, and touch. Consequently, we are perpetually exposed to various environmental toxins, synthetic chemicals, and harmful substances. Luckily for us, our bodies have a remarkable built-in detoxification system to remove these unwanted invaders.

Detoxification is the body's natural process of eliminating or neutralizing toxins through the colon, liver, kidneys, lungs, lymph nodes, and skin. In essence, detoxification transforms these toxins into less harmful compounds that can be safely excreted from the body. Our body performs this intricate process routinely, in two phases: Phase I (modification) and Phase II (conjugation).

In the Phase I detoxification, the liver enzymes, known as Cytochrome P450, work to convert harmful toxins into less harmful substances, albeit they may still be reactive. In the Phase II process, these semi-reactive substances are transformed into water-soluble compounds that can be easily excreted via sweat, urine, or feces.

2.2. Understanding Endogenous and Exogenous Toxins

Toxins that our bodies need to detoxify can be classified into two groups: endogenous and exogenous toxins.

Endogenous toxins are metabolic waste products produced by our body. Some examples are ammonia and lactic acid produced during regular cell activity. Other endogenous toxins include stress-produced hormones like adrenaline or waste from dying or dead cells.

Exogenous toxins are substances that come from our environment. They might be breathed, ingested, absorbed through the skin, or generated through the metabolism of drugs or food additives. Examples include heavy metals (like lead, mercury), exhaust fumes, tobacco smoke, pesticides, household cleaners, and even certain food preservatives.

2.3. Detoxification and Nutrition

Optimal nutrition can enhance the body's detoxification process. Certain nutrients are particularly beneficial, acting as cofactors for the enzymes involved in Phase I and II detoxification.

For instance, B vitamins, minerals like magnesium, and antioxidants such as vitamin C and E are essential for Phase I. In the Phase II, sulfur-containing compounds found in garlic and onions, amino acids like glycine and glutamine, and compounds like glucosinolates found in cruciferous vegetables, can aid the detoxification process.

Protein, particularly from animal source, is also crucial because it supplies the sulfur-containing amino acids necessary for Phase II. However, a balance is necessary as too much protein can also generate ammonia, an endogenous toxin.

2.4. The Myth of Quick Fix Detoxes

Over the last few decades, our understanding of detoxification has been marred by the overwhelming popularity of "quick-fix" detox programs and diets. These supposedly speed up the body's detoxification mechanism and aid in rapid weight loss. However, there is very minimal scientific evidence to support such claims, and they may inadvertently cause harm by encouraging potentially unhealthy behaviors like fasting or excessive nutritional restriction.

Such detox plans often revolve around drastic diet changes, juicing, or the use of detoxifying supplements. It is critical to note that although these may lead to temporary weight loss, it's typically due to water weight and muscle mass reduction rather than actual loss of body fat. Additionally, the focus on reduced calorie intake might lead to nutrient deficiencies, leading to problems like weakened immunity, fatigue, and mood swings.

2.5. Detox and Health: A Balanced Approach

The best approach to support your body's detoxification system is through balanced lifestyle choices: eating a nutrient-dense diet rich in whole foods, maintaining an active life, staying hydrated, getting adequate sleep, and managing stress.

Incorporate a variety of fruits, vegetables, whole grains, lean protein, and healthy fats in your diet to ensure you get a rich supply of detox-aiding nutrients. Exercise regularly to boost your metabolism and help your body eliminate toxins through sweat. Keep yourself well-hydrated to support the regular flushing out of toxins. Prioritize good sleep, as many of our body's detox processes kick in more effectively during sleep.

2.6. The Conclusion: Understanding the Nature of Detoxification

The science of detoxification is complex and ever-evolving. It involves numerous biochemical processes that are influenced by many factors: genetic, environmental, nutritional, and lifestyle-oriented. Understanding this interplay is key to debunking the detox myths that are rampant today.

While certain practices can aid our body's detoxification process, there's no quick fix or magic cleanse that will do the job. Instead, a balanced approach embracing healthy dietary and lifestyle practices is what truly supports our body's innate detox mechanisms, leading to improved well-being and vitality.

The allure of quick and dramatic results can sometimes cloud our judgement; however, true health is a lifelong journey and not a destination to be reached overnight. As we enhance our knowledge, we can make informed choices that support our body in its work and cherish the health benefits that evolve from these decisions over time.

Remember, the path to health is paved with good habits. Invest in understanding your body better to make smart decisions towards a fitter, healthier, and happier YOU!

Chapter 3. Diving into Efficient Training Regimes

If you're a fitness novice or a seasoned athlete, understanding and implementing efficient training regimes is pivotal to achieving sustained results and predominant wellness. This section will provide a comprehensive examination of diverse training regimes, their practical implementation and potential benefits for various fitness levels and goals.

3.1. Understanding the Importance of Training Regimes

A training regimen, sometimes termed as a workout routine or training programme, represents a systematic approach to exercise that consider your fitness goals, present condition, and available resources. These regimes cater to evolving needs, by adopting a multidimensional approach towards fitness – incorporating strength training, cardiovascular training, flexibility activities, and rest periods into one comprehensive pack.

Remember, everyone has distinct fitness needs and preferences, and a training regimen isn't 'one-size-fits-all'. Comprehensive training regimes should be adaptable, challenging, and rewardingly efficacious to keep you motivated and engrossed throughout your fitness journey.

An efficient training regimen can help:

- Improve cardiovascular health

- Sculpt and strengthen muscles

- Improve body composition

- Boost physical endurance and performance

- Enhance flexibility and mobility

- Promote better sleep

- Mitigate stress and anxiety

3.2. Choosing the Right Training Regimen

The first order of business in creating or choosing a training regime is to understand your aim – whether it's to lose fat, build muscle, enhance cardiovascular endurance, augment sports performance, or just improve general health. Consider your current fitness level and time commitment, as this would dictate the intensity and frequency of your regimen.

Here are four scopes of training:

1. HIIT (High-Intensity Interval Training): Notable for speedy and effective fat loss progress, HIIT integrates high-intensity bouts of exercise followed by short recuperation stretches.

Example:

```
Run at a high speed for 1 minute, followed by 2 minutes
of slow walking or resting, and repeat.
```

1. Resistance Training: Predominantly targeted on muscle building and strength improvement. This often involves weightlifting or bodyweight exercises.

Example:

```
3 sets of 10 repetitions of squats, bench presses, and
```

deadlifts, with rest intervals between sets.

1. Circuit Training: An amalgamation of cardio-strength routines executed one after the other with brief interims of rest, providing an all-inclusive workout.

Example:

5 minutes of jogging, followed by 1 set each of lunges, push-ups, jumping jacks, and sit-ups, repeated twice or thrice.

1. Endurance Training: Primarily augments cardiovascular endurance; often comprises low-intensity, long-duration activities.

Example:

Long-distance running, swimming, or cycling for extended periods without rest.

3.3. Putting Your Training Regimen into Action

Structure and consistency are key aspects of implementing a training regimen. After identifying your fitness objectives and viable training method, develop a weekly schedule that incorporates regular exercise, rest, and occasional mix-ups to avoid plateauing and stay engaged.

Consider the 'FITT' principle to design your regimen:

1. Frequency: How often do you plan to train? If you're a beginner, think about starting with 2-3 sessions per week and gradually intensifying.

2. Intensity: How hard will you train? Strive for a balance: pushing yourself towards progress, yet not to the extent of danger or exhaustion.

3. Time: How long will your workouts be? Depending on your regimen, workouts can range from quick 15-minute circuits to hour-long endurance sessions.

4. Type: What type of workout will you be doing? Incorporate strength, cardio, and flexibility exercises for a holistic regime.

Here's a sample weekly schedule based on FITT:

```
- Monday: 1 hour of resistance training (Medium
Intensity)
- Tuesday: 30 minutes of HIIT (High Intensity)
- Wednesday: Rest
- Thursday: 1 hour of endurance training (Low Intensity)
- Friday: 30 minutes of circuit training (Medium-High
Intensity)
- Saturday: Rest or optional stretching/flexibility
session
- Sunday: Rest
```

Remember, listening to your body's cues is vital – adaptation and flexibility are often the unspoken success factors in any training regimen. Honor rest days, balanced nutrition, and adequate hydration along with your compound training to facilitate the desired transformation effectively.

Achieving fitness goals takes time and patience; so, stay persistent, enjoy each workout, and soon, you'll witness the physical and mental changes that come with a mindful, rightly directed training regimen!

Chapter 4. Power up: Building a Nutritional Plan that Works

In the pursuit of fitness, a formidable ally is having a solid and individualized nutritional plan. This can make the difference between meeting fitness goals and falling short. Here, we delve into the details of designing a plan that's fun, flexible, and completely feasible.

4.1. I. Understanding Nutrition

Before creating a nutrition plan that works, it's important to have a grasp of the basics of nutrition. Nutrition impacts a wide spectrum of physical and mental functions, from supplying the body with energy to supporting brain function.

Macronutrients; proteins, carbohydrates and fats are the substances our bodies need in large amounts. Simply put: * Proteins are the building blocks of your muscles, skin, enzymes, and hormones and are essential for growth and repair. * Carbohydrates are your body's main source of energy: they help fuel your brain, kidneys, heart, muscles and central nervous system. * Fats are a major source of energy, assist in nutrient absorption, and protect your heart and brain health.

Besides these, micronutrients; vitamins and minerals, are essential but in smaller quantities. They are crucial for the production of enzymes, hormones, and other substances that help development and disease prevention.

4.2. II. Assessing Your Dietary Needs

Your nutritional needs will depend on several factors, like age, gender, weight, height, and physical activity levels. A young, physically active male will require a different nutritional plan than an older, sedentary female.

You can utilize online calculators or registered dietitians to help determine your calorie and macro needs. Remember to set realistic and timely goals for yourself, rather than setting unrealistic and difficult to achieve targets.

4.3. III. Building Your Nutritional Plan

Once you've understood your dietary needs, it's time to create your nutritional plan.

1. **Balance is Key** Diversify your diet to include a variety of foods from all food groups in the right proportions. Each meal should ideally contain a source of protein, complex carbohydrates, and healthy fats.

2. **Portion Control** Use measuring cups, kitchen scales, or visual estimates to ensure you're consuming the right amount of food.

3. **Menu Planning** Having a plan removes the stress of deciding what to eat at each meal and reduces the temptations to cheat on your diet.

4. **Stay Hydrated** Water is essential for various bodily functions and good health. It helps remove waste, regulate body temperature, and provide cushioning for joints.

4.4. IV. Foods to Include and Excluded Foods

Emphasizing fresh, whole foods while minimizing processed items is a good rule of thumb.

Foods to Include:

- High quality proteins: Lean meats, poultry, fish, eggs, tofu, and legumes
- Complex carbohydrates: Whole grains, fruits, vegetables
- Healthy fats: Avocados, nuts, seeds, olive oil, fatty fish
- Micronutrients: Choose a rainbow of fruits and vegetables

Excluded Foods:

- Processed foods: Chips, cookies, ready meals, fast food.
- Refined sugars: Sweetened drinks, candies, pastries.
- Unhealthy fats: Trans fats, high-fat meat, high-fat dairy, coconut and palm oil.

4.5. V. Meal Timing and Frequency

Lastly, don't overlook the timing of your meals. Regular eating intervals can prevent overeating, maintain blood sugar levels and aid metabolic functions. This doesn't mandate a rigid five-meal regimen, but rather listening to your body signals and ensuring nourishment throughout the day.

4.6. VI. Sustainability

Make your nutritional plan one that you can stick to. It should not feel overly restrictive and should fit in with your lifestyle. Remember, it is not about a quick fix but making long-term changes. A sustainable plan is always more effective for maintaining fitness goals.

Remember, you deserve a plan that works for you. Every body is unique, and what works for one person may not work for you. So listen to your body and adjust your nutritional plan as necessary. Now, put this knowledge into action and power up your health, one meal at a time.

Chapter 5. The Symbiotic Relationship between Diet and Exercise

A healthy lifestyle involves more than just exercise or eating right; it is about understanding and embodying the intricate, symbiotic relationship between the two. Exercising regularly while also maintaining a balanced diet can do wonders for you physically, psychologically, and emotionally.

5.1. Nutrition: The Building Blocks of Fitness

The foundation of a healthy lifestyle is good nutrition. Food fuels our bodies, providing vital energy and nutrients necessary for various bodily processes, including muscle recovery, cell regeneration, brain function, and immune response. That's why what you consume not only affects your weight but your overall wellbeing, energy levels, and athletic performance.

When it comes to exercise, your body needs certain nutrients before and after a workout for optimal performance and recovery. Regular consumption of macronutrients (carbohydrates, proteins, fats) as well as micronutrients (vitamins and minerals) is key.

Carbohydrates provide valuable glucose, stored as glycogen in the muscles and liver, which acts as our principal energy source during moderate to high-intensity workouts. In contrast, fats are the primary fuel for lower-intensity activities. Protein intake is crucial for muscle repair and growth after a workout.

Micro-nutrient needs depend on many factors, including your type and level of physical activity and overall health. Minerals like Iron, Zinc, Calcium, and Magnesium, along with vitamins such as A, B, C, D, E, and K, are invaluable to both maintaining health and optimizing physical performance.

5.2. Impact of Nutrition on Athletic Performance

A balanced diet is integral to achieving your fitness goals, regardless of whether they involve running a marathon, lifting heavier weights, or increasing your flexibility. Without proper nutrition, your body can't perform at its peak, making it harder for you to achieve your fitness goals.

Your body needs dietary proteins to repair and build tissues, including muscles. Since exercise puts stress on bodily tissues, causing them to break down and inflammation to occur, eating a protein-rich meal after workout assists in muscle recovery and growth.

Carbohydrates are king for endurance athletes. Consuming whole grains, fruits, and vegetables provides a slow-release energy source that can help you push through long workout sessions. For optimum performance during intense training, athletes should ensure they consume enough carbohydrates to maintain their glycogen stores.

Even hydration plays a significant role in athletic performance. Dehydration can lead to muscle cramps, dizziness, and fatigue – some of the primary performance killers. Thus, drinking adequate water before, during, and after your training is crucial.

5.3. Exercise: The Catalyst for Optimal Nutrition

While nutrition forms the core of a healthy lifestyle, exercise acts as a catalyst, enhancing nutrition absorption, and optimizing its benefits on bodily functions and systems.

Exercise is known to stimulate muscle contractions, thereby enhancing the absorption of glucose and amino acids, which leads to increased muscle protein synthesis, improved insulin sensitivity, and better blood sugar management. It also hastens the transit of food in the gut, improving digestion and nutrient absorption.

Moreover, regular physical activity can influence dietary habits. Research shows that people become more conscious of their food choices after exercise, gravitating towards healthier food options and maintaining better portion control.

Exercise also plays a critical role in maintaining a healthy body weight. A balance between caloric intake and expenditure is necessary for weight management. Regular exercise can increase your metabolic rate, helping you burn more calories and possibly influence your appetite and food choices.

5.4. The Cycle: How Diet and Exercise Influence Each Other

The synergy between diet and exercise is so profound that changes in one can substantially impact the other. For example, if you switch from a sedentary lifestyle to regular, intense workouts, your nutritional needs will shift dramatically. Conversely, adopting a diet low in nutrients and high in processed foods can hinder your ability to exercise effectively, leading to fatigue, slow recovery, and even injury.

Creating the right synergy starts with understanding your fitness goals and how different types of exercise influence your body's nutritional needs. For instance, resistance or strength training requires higher protein to assist with muscle repair and building, while endurance training necessitates replenished carbohydrate stores.

The link between diet and exercise also extends to meal timing, with research indicating that when you eat matters just as much as what you eat. Eating something small and carbohydrate-rich before workouts can provide a quick energy source, while consuming protein post-workout aids in muscle recovery.

In summary, the partnership of a balanced diet and regular exercise is vital for achieving your health and fitness goals and maintaining long-term wellness. While diet provides the necessary fuel, exercise triggers body mechanisms to utilize these nutrients optimally. This symbiotic relationship between diet and exercise underlines the importance of harmonizing the two to lead a sustainable, healthy lifestyle.

Chapter 6. Mastering the Art of Smart Eating

A sound dietary regime is the cornerstone of a vital and healthy life. With a flux of unregulated dietary information, making smart eating choices can often seem overwhelming. However, by understanding the fundamentals, you can equip yourself with the knowledge to devise a dietary plan that is both nutritionally complete and satisfying.

6.1. The Building Blocks of Nutrition

At their core, all foods are composed of three macronutrients – carbohydrates, proteins, and fats. An understanding of these macronutrients and how they function in your body is crucial for smart eating.

Carbohydrates are the main source of quick energy for the body. Simple carbohydrates found in refined sugars and fruits are quickly absorbed, while complex carbohydrates in whole grains and vegetables are digested more slowly.

Proteins are the building blocks of the body. They play a crucial role in muscle development and repair, hormone production, and numerous other bodily functions. Sources of protein include meat, dairy, fish, and plant-based proteins like lentils and chickpeas.

Fats are a concentrated source of energy and are essential for several bodily functions, including vitamin absorption and hormone regulation. Unsaturated fats found in olive oil, avocados, and fish offer various health benefits, whereas trans and saturated fats in processed food can lead to numerous health challenges.

6.2. Balance is Key: Understanding the Nutritional Plate

For smart eating, developing balanced meals is critical. The nutritional plate serves as a visual guide for composing such meals. Envision your plate divided into four sections.

- Half of the plate should be filled with a variety of fruits and vegetables, providing rich sources of vitamins, minerals, and fiber.

- One quarter of the plate should be allocated to lean proteins.

- The remaining quarter should contain whole grains or starchy vegetables to provide necessary complex carbohydrates.

- Lastly, incorporate some form of healthy fat into each meal such as avocado or a drizzle of olive oil.

6.3. Making Informed Choices: Navigating the Supermarket

Often the foods marketed as 'healthy' are anything but. Understanding food labeling is crucial to supplement your smart eating plan. Here are few tips for you:

- Read beyond the front label. Don't be swayed by health claims on the front of the package. Instead, always check the nutritional label and ingredient list.

- Look out for hidden sugars. Ingredients ending in 'ose', such as fructose or sucrose, are forms of sugar.

- Choose foods low in saturated fats, sodium, and added sugars.

- Opt for whole, unprocessed foods whenever possible.

6.4. Beyond the Basics: The Power of Superfoods

Certain foods, often branded as 'superfoods', contain a higher-than-average quantity of beneficial nutrients. These include antioxidant-rich berries, nutrient-dense leafy greens, omega-3-rich chia seeds, and more. Integrating such foods can add an extra nutritional punch to your meals.

6.5. The Role of Hydration

Water is essential for life. Staying well-hydrated aids digestion, nutrient absorption, waste elimination, and overall metabolic function. Aim for eight 8-ounce glasses, about 2 liters, or half a gallon of water a day.

6.6. Tailoring Your Diet to Your Training

Your dietary needs would shift depending on your exercise routine, intensity, and duration. It's necessary to fuel workouts with enough carbohydrates and proteins. Likewise, consuming a protein-rich meal within an hour post-workout aids in muscle recovery.

By adopting these principles, you're well on your way to mastering the art of smart eating. This journey will guide you toward optimum health, improved bodily function, and a revitalized sense of well-being.

Chapter 7. Gearing up: Choosing the Right Equipment for your Fitness Journey

Getting started on a fitness journey is an exciting endeavor, bringing the promise of improved health, vitality and well-being. Whether you are a complete beginner or an avid fitness enthusiast, having the right gear and equipment can make all the difference. This chapter will guide you through the process of selecting appropriate fitness equipment that aligns with your goals and promotes a safe, effective exercise routine.

7.1. Understanding Your Fitness Goals

Your fitness goals are an essential starting point when choosing your workout equipment. Are you looking to lose weight? Enhance overall fitness? Maybe you aim to improve cardio health or boost strength? Determining your goals will provide a roadmap for the equipment that will best assist your journey.

For weight loss and cardio health, consider equipment that facilitates aerobic activity such as treadmills, stationary bikes or elliptical trainers. For muscle building and strength, resistive equipment like weight machines, free weights, and kettlebells are effective.

7.2. Safety First – Protecting Your Body

Equally as critical as the exercise equipment, protective gear is fundamental to injury prevention. This encompasses everything from the right shoes supporting your foot type and training style to clothing that allows maximum flexibility and minimal chafing.

Shoes: Different training types require specific shoes that provide unique support and shield you from injury. Running shoes provide shock absorption critical for high-impact activities, while cross-training shoes provide lateral support suited for gym or mid-level impact workouts.

Workout clothes: Look for moisture-wicking fabrics that keep sweat off your skin reducing friction and irritation. Ensure your clothing allows ample movement for your specific workouts.

Other protective gear may include gloves, helmets, padding, or goggles, depending on your fitness activity.

7.3. The Right Gear for a Home Workout

Home workouts offer convenience and flexibility, but they require space-efficient and versatile equipment. Resistance bands and adjustable dumbbells are adaptable for a range of workouts and easily storable. Foldable treadmills and exercise bikes are also popular options.

Online resources can guide you on setting up a home workout area effectively to avoid the upfront cost and ongoing fees of gym memberships.

7.4. Upgrading Your Cardio: Treadmill, Elliptical, or Stationary Bike?

Cardiovascular equipment is central to any fitness journey geared towards weight management, stamina improvement, and overall health.

Treadmills simulate natural running and walking movements making it easy to use. The adjustable speed and incline offer a range of difficulty levels.

Elliptical trainers or cross trainers create a fluid motion that is low on joint impact, ideal for elderly exercisers or those with joint problems.

On the other hand, stationary bikes provide effective lower body and cardio workouts in a seated position, making it less impactful on joints and suitable for all fitness levels.

7.5. Building Strength: Free Weights, Machines, or Both?

Strength training is a crucial component of a well-rounded fitness regime. Free weights engage more muscles, enhancing balance and fostering functional fitness. They include barbells, dumbbells, kettlebells, and medicine balls.

Weight machines focus on isolated muscle groups, reducing the risk of injury and allowing for greater weight load. They are useful for beginners or rehabilitating individuals.

Most experts will agree that a combination of both is optimal, allowing for a balanced, comprehensive strength program that promotes muscle symmetry and reduces injury risk.

7.6. Tech Tools and Fitness Apps

Merging technology with fitness has produced a suite of tools that track, motivate, and guide you towards your fitness goals. Fitness trackers monitor key data points like steps, heart rate, and calories burned, providing meaningful insights into your progress.

Fitness apps offer vast resources, from guided workouts and meal planning to virtual coaching, making them a helpful investment in your fitness journey.

In conclusion, choosing the right equipment for your fitness journey is essential in ensuring that your exercises are effective and safe. A clear understanding of your fitness goals, awareness of comfort and safety, and the power of selection can significantly impact your journey's success and enjoyment. Remember, the best equipment is the one that you will use consistently. Invest wisely in pieces that you enjoy and suit your unique fitness goals.

Chapter 8. Creating a Personalised Fitness Schedule

The journey towards optimal health and fitness begins with clear, personalized goals and a schedule tailored to meet them. Remember, every person is unique. What works for one individual may not necessarily work for another. Ensuring you're pursuing a fitness regime that respects your lifestyle, preferences, physical condition, and long-term goals can mean the difference between success and frustration.

8.1. Understanding Your Fitness Goals

Before you begin drawing up your personal fitness schedule, it's essential to establish your fitness goals. Whether it's losing weight, gaining muscle, improving cardio health, increasing flexibility, boosting stamina or a combination of these, a clear vision will act as a roadmap as you chart your fitness journey.

Define your fitness goals based on the SMART principle, i.e., they should be Specific, Measurable, Attainable, Relevant, and Time-bound. A poorly thought-out objective such as "I want to get fit" is too vague. Instead, translate it into SMART terms, such as "I want to lose 20 pounds within the next four months."

8.2. Assess Your Current Fitness Level

Before we dive into the heart of your training schedule, let's take a moment to assess your current fitness level. You can get a rough gauge by asking yourself how much physical activity you usually engage in each week. Physical exams, such as heart rate check before and after exercising, can be beneficial, as well as strength and endurance assessments.

It's critical to consult a medical professional or a certified fitness professional for a thorough health check-up before beginning any new fitness program. They can help determine your fitness level, potential health risks and advise you on any precautions you should take.

8.3. Knowing Your Schedule

A crucial aspect of creating a personalized fitness schedule involves examining your daily timetable. Realistically assess how much time you can allocate to your fitness regime. Be honest with yourself. If your work or family commitments don't allow you to spend two hours at the gym every day, there's no point forcing it.

Think about when you want to work out - in the morning, at lunch, or after work? The best time to work out is whenever you can make it a consistent part of your schedule. Research suggests that both morning and evening workouts can provide unique benefits, so choose a time that suits you best.

8.4. Establish a mix of exercises

There's no one-size-fits-all approach to exercise. Your workout routine should include a mix of cardiovascular exercise (like walking, running, or cycling), strength training (like weight lifting), flexibility exercises (like yoga), and balance exercises. This balanced mix can help to prevent workout boredom, offer a full body workout, and reduce the risk of injury.

Cardiovascular exercises promote heart health and endurance, strength training will help in building lean muscle mass, flexibility exercises to keep the muscles supple and to improve your range of motion, and balance exercises for stability.

Tailor your mix based on your fitness level and goals. For instance, if your goal is to build muscle, you'll want to put more emphasis on strength training.

8.5. Sample Weekly Workout Schedule

Creating a weekly workout schedule ensures that you have a well-rounded routine. You are more likely to stick with it over the long term. Below is an example of what a weekly schedule might look like:

1. A sample week for beginners:
    - Monday: 30 minutes of moderate cardio
    - Tuesday: 20 minutes of weight/strength training
    - Wednesday: Rest
    - Thursday: 20 minutes of weight/strength training
    - Friday: 30 minutes of moderate cardio
    - Saturday: Rest
    - Sunday: 30 minutes of weight training

2. A sample week for intermediate/advanced:
    - Monday: 30 minutes of high-intensity interval training (HIIT)
    - Tuesday: 45 minutes of weight/strength training
    - Wednesday: 30 minutes of moderate-intensity cardio plus balance exercises
    - Thursday: 45 minutes of weight/strength training

- Friday: 30 minutes of HIIT

- Saturday: 45 minutes of weight/strength training

- Sunday: Rest

8.6. Making Adjustments

Keep in mind, this fitness schedule is not static. Adjustments might become necessary as your body changes, or as you progress and your goals evolve. Additionally, it's absolutely essential to listen to your body. If you're feeling overly tired or you're in pain, take an extra rest day. There's no harm in resting; in fact, your body needs recovery time to heal, grow stronger and to avoid injury.

Having your workout schedule in place, you are ready for your fitness journey. It's your ticket to health, happiness, and a fitter version of yourself. So, don your gym wear and get started on your personalized fitness schedule today! And remember - consistency is key. It's not about perfection; it's about effort. And when you bring that effort every single day, that's where transformation happens.

Chapter 9. The Role of Hydration in Detox and Training

Water is the most fundamental element for our survival. Without it, digestion, absorption, circulation, and excretion – all key bodily functions – would be impossible. It only makes sense, then, to begin our discussion about detoxification and training by addressing the role of hydration.

9.1. The connection between hydration and detoxification

Detoxification is a natural process that takes place in our body to expel waste and toxic substances. The primary actors in this process are our liver and kidneys, which work to purify our bloodstream. Keeping these organs adequately hydrated is integral to enabling them to carry out their vital detoxification functions.

Water helps our kidneys by diluting and expelling toxins in the urine. Dehydration can strain these vital organs, impede their ability to filter waste, and elevate the risk of kidney stones.

Similarly, the liver, one of the body's primary detoxification organs, requires water to convert toxins into water-soluble substances which can be excreted from the body more easily.

Additionally, water aids in digestion. It assists in breaking down food to extract nutrients and serves as a vehicle to move insoluble wastes through the intestines for elimination.

9.2. The relationship between hydration and training

Hydration is equally crucial for those engaging in physical exercise. During a workout, our bodies heat up, we sweat to cool down, losing fluids and essential electrolytes in the process. This loss must be replenished to maintain a healthy balance, prevent dehydration, and maintain peak physical performance.

When the body is dehydrated, blood thickens, forcing the heart to work harder to pump blood and provide oxygen and nutrients to muscles. Also, water is required for muscle contractions, and any shortage can lead to muscle cramping and stiffness.

Further, drinking water before, during, and after workouts aids in preventing fatigue, maintains energy levels, facilitates recovery, and often improves overall performance.

9.3. Hydration recommendations for detox and training

The "eight glasses a day" rule is a useful starting point for understanding how much water we need, but it does not consider individual factors like physical activity, body size, and climate.

For those engaging in moderate to intense workouts, sports medicine specialists recommend drinking a combination of water and sports drinks. The latter replenishes electrolytes lost through sweat. A good rule of thumb is to drink 2-3 cups of water 2-3 hours before exercise, and about 1 cup every 15-20 minutes during the workout.

As for detox purposes, other fluid sources like herbal teas, fresh fruit and vegetable juices, or detox water enriched with sliced fruits, mint, or cinnamon can be a great addition to your hydration routine.

9.4. Hydration and longevity

Scientific evidence suggests a link between hydration and longevity. Studies show that cells that stay hydrated are better at fighting off diseases and staying healthy. Hydrated cells are more efficient in absorbing nutrients and expelling waste.

In summary, maintaining proper hydration is vital for detoxification, training, and overall well-being. It empowers your body to function smoothly, fosters peak physical performance, aids in proper waste elimination, and can even contribute to a longer, healthier life. It's the simplest but one of the most effective steps towards a fitter, healthier, and happier YOU!

It's important to remember that individual needs vary, and it's crucial to listen to your body. Signs such as feeling thirsty, dark yellow urine, headaches, or feeling tired can often indicate that your body needs more water.

In the coming chapters, we'll delve deeper into other key elements of detox and training, including diet, exercise routines, sleep, and the role of mindset. Keep reading, stay hydrated, and remember – every small step can contribute to large health gains!

That being said, water alone is not a magic fix. Hydration should be balanced with a nutritious diet, adequate sleep, regular exercise, and a positive mindset to achieve a wholesome reboot. It's imperative not to view it in isolation but as an integral part of a holistic wellness strategy. It's also worth noting that while water supports detoxification, it doesn't 'detox' in the sense of removing toxins that the body would not have otherwise removed.

Chapter 10. Mental Health: Essential Player in Your Fitness Journey

Understanding the critical role of mental health in the fitness journey is a nuanced and broad topic. The interplay between mental health and physical health is deep-seated and significantly affects not only the way you perceive fitness but also how you engage in and benefit from physical activities.

10.1. Comprehensive Overview of Mental Health

Mental health refers to more than the absence of mental health conditions or illnesses. It is an integral part of health as declared by the World Health Organization (WHO): "Health is not merely the absence of disease or infirmity but complete physical, mental and social wellbeing." It pertains to our feelings, how we think, and how we behave. It influences how we manage stress, relate to others, and make choices. Mental health is pivotal at every stage of life, from childhood and adolescence through adulthood.

Mental health disorders that often come to mind include anxiety disorders, mood disorders, psychotic disorders, eating disorders, trauma-related disorders, and substance abuse disorders. This chapter will focus on the relationship between these mental health conditions and fitness, but remember that preserving and boosting mental health in the broader sense is also a vital aspect of your fitness journey.

10.2. Connection between Physical Fitness and Mental Health

Exercise has long been recognized for its beneficial effects on mental health. Research has found that physical activity can help alleviate symptoms associated with mild to moderate depression and anxiety. Regular exercise also relieves stress, improves memory, helps with sleep, and boosts overall mood.

When you exercise, your body releases chemicals called endorphins. These endorphins interact with the receptors in your brain that reduce your perception of pain. Endorphins also trigger a positive feeling in the body, similar to that of morphine.

Beyond the "feel-good" effect, regular physical activity can increase self-confidence, improve body image, and decrease symptoms related with mild depression and anxiety. Exercise can also help improve cognitive function and decreases the risk of death from suicide.

10.3. Impact of Mental Health on Physical Fitness

While the beneficial impacts of physical fitness on mental health are well established, it's equally vital to recognize that mental health significantly influences physical fitness. Mental health conditions, especially when untreated or poorly managed, can interfere with one's ability or motivation to engage in physical activities. For instance, depression or anxiety can lead to decreased energy levels, and this fatigue or apathy may present as a major barrier to initiating or maintaining an exercise routine.

Furthermore, substance abuse disorders can lead to severe health issues, including cardiovascular diseases, which could further hinder physical fitness. It is therefore crucial to adequately address these problems and seek professional help if needed. Your mental and emotional health is key to maintaining your routines and achieving your fitness goals.

10.4. Strategies to Improve Mental Health in Your Fitness Journey

10.4.1. Engagement is Key

Identify physical activities that you enjoy, such as dancing, gardening, hiking, or biking, and integrate these activities into your exercise routine. The more you enjoy an activity, the easier it is to make it a part of your everyday schedule.

10.4.2. Set Realistic Goals

Setting achievable fitness goals can also contribute to mental health. Whether you're aiming to lose weight, tone muscles, improve endurance, or increase flexibility, be sure to set realistic and manageable goals.

10.4.3. Regular Relaxation and Stress Management

Techniques such as deep breathing, mediation, yoga, and tai chi can help decrease stress and anxiety, making it easier to incorporate regular exercise into your routine. These practices are also a good way to warm up or cool down around your main exercise routine.

10.5. Implementing a Holistic Approach

A holistic approach to health is one that considers mental and physical wellbeing as integrated and inseparable. By taking care of your mental health and using it as a springboard for physical health, you'll be primed to reach greater levels of fitness and everyday well-being. Similarly, by keeping a solid focus on your physical health and fitness activities, you can boost your mental health and build psychological resilience. It's like a positive feedback loop that leads to a healthier, happier you.

Indeed, mental health isn't just an "add-on" to your fitness journey. It's a critical player - a driving force, motivator, and ingredient for long-term success.

Chapter 11. Keeping the Momentum: Tips for Long-term Fitness Commitment

A fitness journey must be recognized as a long-term lifestyle change rather than a short-lived project. While starting a new fitness regime can come with an initial burst of motivation and enthusiasm, the real challenge lies in maintaining the momentum.

11.1. Understanding the Importance of Consistency

Any fitness journey begins with setting clear, realistic goals. But what actually propels you toward these goals is the consistency of effort and commitment. Regularity in exercise fosters an improved range of motion, strength, endurance, and overall physical function.

During the first days and weeks of your training, you may not observe significant changes. However, consistency over the long term pays off generously, leading to noticeable progress in performance and changes in the mirror. Commitment to your routine, irrespective of the ups and downs of life, is the key ingredient to reaping optimal health benefits.

11.2. Confronting and Overcoming Obstacles

You will face inevitable obstacles on your journey - scheduling conflicts, lack of motivation, injuries, or even plateaus in your progress. It's essential to recognize these hurdles as part and parcel of the journey, and not as reasons to quit.

When life gets in the way, and it eventually will, you could try shortening your workout instead of skipping it altogether or replace vigorous workouts with light activities. In case of injuries, consult your healthcare professional and seek advice on revisions for your workout regime.

Lack of motivation can be a tricky hurdle to navigate. Try to identify the root cause—whether it's boredom, fatigue, or stress—and address it accordingly. You could switch up your workouts or workout times, engage in fun physical activities, or even join a fitness group to maintain your interest.

11.3. Strategies to Foster Persistence

A few strategies could help maintain your momentum when it starts to dwindle:

- **Set SMART Goals**: SMART (Specific, Measurable, Achievable, Relevant, Time-bound) goals provide direction and motivation. They keep you driven, provide a track to progress, and facilitate realistic expectations.

- **Plan Your Schedule**: Pre-plan your workouts weekly and treat them as non-negotiable appointments. Preparation reduces stress and odds of missed workouts, hence boosting consistency.

- **Keep it Enjoyable**: If you dread it, you'll probably avoid it. Make sure your fitness routine involves exercises that you love, or mix things up by trying new workouts.

- **Celebrate Progress**: Recognize and celebrate when you reach a milestone. This could be as simple as treating yourself to a new pair of running shoes or signing up for advanced training.

11.4. The Role of Nutrition in Long-Term Fitness Commitment

Fitness and nutrition have a symbiotic relationship; one complements and enhances the other. While your workouts help you stay fit, how you fuel your body plays an equally important part in the process. The key is to find a balanced diet that works for you, filled with natural, nutrient-dense foods that provide the energy you need.

Establishing a healthy eating pattern not only nourishes your body to withstand physically demanding workouts but also supports faster recovery. Proper nutrition ensures your metabolism is operative, helping you shed fat and build muscle. Neglecting this aspect might lead to energy crashes, slower progress, and increased risk of injury, eventually hampering your overall fitness commitment.

11.5. Conclusion

Staying committed to long-term fitness is a marathon, not a sprint. Perseverance, patience, and consistency are the qualities that will see you through. Remember, there's no one-size-fits-all approach to fitness. Recognize and respect your unique body, its limitations, and potential. Listen to your body, prioritize rest and recovery, and make regular health check-ups part of your routine.

Most importantly, render your fitness journey a part of your lifestyle, rather than a burdensome task to check off your daily list.

Embrace the journey wholeheartedly, not just the destination, and you'll find that staying committed to long-term fitness becomes a natural, enjoyably intrinsic part of your life.

www.ingramcontent.com/pod-product-compliance
Lightning Source LLC
Chambersburg PA
CBHW071043260726

48661CB00007B/3126